Cognitive Implications of Dementia: A Caregiver's Guide to Improve Communication and Swallow Function

Christina M. Freise MS CCC-SLP, CBIS

Text by Christina M. Freise, copyright 2017

All rights reserved. No part of this publication may be reproduced, distributed or transmitted in any form or by any means, or stored in a database or retrieval system, without the prior written permission from the copyright owner.

First e-book edition 2017
First paperback edition 2018

Introduction

Thank you so very much for purchasing this book. I hope that you find the tools within this book to transform your interactions with your loved one with dementia. This book is not meant to replace an evaluation and treatment by a physician or speech-language pathologist; it is meant to provide you, the caregiver, with practical information to communicate effectively with your loved one. I hope you find the suggestions and activities to follow highly beneficial in your communicative interactions and during mealtime. If you have any constructive feedback to improve the content of this book, please email me at info@speechbythebeach.org, as I am always looking to refine my work and please my readers.

About the author:
Christina Freise is a Speech-Language Pathologist and Certified Brain Injury Specialist, holding a Masters of Science in Speech-Language Pathology from Columbia University, New York, New York. Her diverse experiences include acute care assessment and management in a Level I Trauma Center, long-term acute care, university clinical faculty member, and owner of *Speech By The Beach Consulting LLC*, a private concierge practice in Naples, Florida. Ms. Freise is the President of the Collier County Medical Society Alliance, a non-profit organization that provides college scholarships to high school students interested in medical careers. She resides in Naples, Florida with her rescue dogs, Bentley and Coco.

Acknowledgements

I was never good at "making things" in the traditional sense of the phrase. My high school carpentry class performance was lackluster. I remember I whittled some sort of jewelry box: did not really open properly, closed in a cock-eyed manner, and was just completely deformed. I'm really a complete failure, I thought.

But, in the symbolic sense, I think we do need to look outside of the traditional 'box' at our skills. So, in the pages that follow is my own box of sorts. It is a box that is filled with passion for the field of speech-language pathology. It is a box that is filled with sincere love and respect for other people, particularly geriatrics. I hope it helps you find what is in your box that makes you a unique gift to society.

A sincere thank you to my former, current, and future patients, as well as their lovely families. You are a daily source of inspiration for me.

Thank you to Dr. Allison Haskill for her time in reviewing this manuscript prior to publication, and for her constant support.

No one has been more instrumental in the pursuit of this project than the members of my family. Thank you to my parents, Maria and Steve, as well as my brother, Patrick, for their love.

A special thank you to my rescue dogs Bentley and Coco for sitting on my lap the entire time I was working on this book.

Please continue to be advocates for those without voices of their own.

Do not ask me to remember,
Don't try to make me understand,
Let me rest and know you're with me,
Kiss my cheek and hold my hand.
I'm confused beyond your concept,
I am sad and sick and lost.
All I know is that I need you
To be with me at all cost.
Do not lose your patience with me,
Do not scold or curse or cry.
I can't help the way I'm acting,
Can't be different though I try.
Just remember that I need you,
That the best of me is gone,
Please don't fail to stand beside me,
Love me 'til my life is done.

– Owen Darnell

What is a Cognitive Communication Impairment?

A cognitive communication impairment is diagnosed when a patient demonstrates any difficulty with communication that is affected by disruption in memory, attention, organization, problem solving, reasoning, and/or executive functions. The most common causes of cognitive communication impairment are the following:

- Stroke
- Traumatic Brain Injury
- Anoxia
- Genetic brain disorders
- Brain Tumor
- Multiple Sclerosis
- Parkinson's disease
- Dementias

This book focuses on cognitive communication impairments that are acquired due to aging, primarily the dementias. Alzheimer's disease is the most common form of dementia, however it is important to note there are other types of dementia including vascular dementia, dementia with Lewy bodies, and frontotemporal dementia.

This book begins with a questionnaire. Please attempt to answer each question as honestly as possible, as it will provide a more accurate stage score. Each person progresses through the stages very differently, and at different rates, thus you may feel the need to re-administer the questionnaire periodically. Please bear in mind that neurologists, neuropsychologists and speech-language pathologists are the experts in cognitive communication deficits. If you are seeking a comprehensive evaluation, please consider visiting one of these professionals.

Cognitive Communication Impairment Questionnaire

Choose the best item below to best describe your loved one. There may not be an option that describes your loved one perfectly, but please select the item closest to the behavior you have witnessed.

* This tool is not meant to be utilized as a substitute to a comprehensive evaluation by a neurologist, neuropsychologist or a speech-language pathologist. It is simply to be utilized as a guide for assisting your loved one. *

1. If you ask your loved one, "What time of day is it?" he/she would respond
   0. With the appropriate time consistently
   1. Generally correct with time of day, however may be 2-3 hours off
   2. Frequently confused about time of day
   3. Rarely knows the time of day
   4. Unable to verbalize or indicate the time of day

2. If you ask your loved one, "Where are we?" when you are at home, he/she would respond:
   0. With the appropriate address consistently
   1. Generally correct, however may be slightly off in terms of numerical detail (i.e. house number error, zip code error)

2. Can name city or state, but cannot recall street name and/or house number
3. Rarely can name a portion of address
4. Unable to verbalize or indicate address

3. In a typical conversation with your loved one, he/she
   0. Can converse typically, asking and answering questions without effort
   1. Engages in typical conversations, but does have times when he/she cannot find a word here or there
   2. Substitutes words for other words, or makes up nonsense words but generally conversation does make sense
   3. Frequently, conversation does not make sense and he/she has difficulty following commands
   4. Unable to verbalize words

4. When eating a meal, your loved one:
   0. Can prepare all meals using recipes, and can feed himself/herself
   1. Can prepare simple meals only such as sandwiches or cereal, and can feed himself/herself
   2. Cannot prepare simple meals, requires some assistance to cut meats, but can feed himself/herself
   3. Needs assistance to feed himself or herself, or frequent reminders to pick up spoon/fork, eat more
   4. Unable to feed self. May note coughing during the meal.

5. When traveling to a given location, your loved one:

0. Has no difficulty navigating (may use a GPS system, map or cane/walker/motorized wheelchair)
1. Can become confused when driving to a new place, even with GPS/maps.
2. Cannot travel to new locations alone safely, but can navigate to familiar locations
3. Can navigate around the house well, but is not trusted to walk around outside
4. Little or no ability to navigate around the home

6. In regards to remembering the names of people, your loved one:
    0. Typically remembers the names of both unfamiliar and familiar people he/she has met
    1. Can forget the names of people he/she has met very few times, but consistently remembers names of familiar people
    2. Can remember children and spouse's names, but cannot remember other names
    3. Can remember spouse or caregiver's name, but cannot remember children's names
    4. Cannot address any person by name

7. When asked questions about his/her personal history, your loved one:
    0. Can state biographical information with great detail
    1. Can provide a general timeline of events in life, but details are vague
    2. Can recall a few events (may be out of sequence) with little/no detail
    3. Recalls one event, may perseverate on this event

4. Does not verbalize any elements of personal history

8. In regards to reading, your loved one:
   0. Reads as he/she did in the past
   1. Reads, but does lose interest faster (may not finish a book or finish the paper)
   2. Reads, but when asked what was read can only provide very rudimentary summary
   3. Will often hold a book or newspaper, but unclear if he/she is actually reading the item.
   4. Does not pick up items with printed words and focus on them in any fashion

9. In regards to counting, your loved one:
   0. Can complete basic finances independently
   1. Requires some assistance for finances (for example, writing a check to pay a bill, but can count change accurately)
   2. All finances must be taken care of by someone else, but he/she can count backwards by 2's from 20, or backwards from 40 by 4's.
   3. Can count from 1-10, but cannot count backwards by 2's from 20
   4. Does not show awareness of numbers or counting

10. When discussing the issues you have observed, your loved one:
    0. I never had this discussion as I haven't noted any issues
    1. Is aware of changes in memory (i.e. misplaces keys), but readily will discuss these changes

2. Often denies changes in cognition, but at times will show awareness (will say, "Maybe I should not be driving anymore.")
3. Completely denies changes in cognition. Makes excuses when he/she forgets something ("I'm just tired").
4. Unable to discuss these changes, completely unaware

Total Score: _____

Scoring Guide:

0: No cognitive communication impairment
1-4: Very mild cognitive decline
5-15: Mild cognitive communication impairment
16-30: Moderate cognitive communication impairment
31-40: Severe cognitive communication impairment

Very Mild Cognitive Decline

(Scores 1-4)

Description of Stage:
This stage is best encapsulated by the term "forgetfulness." Typically, this stage is characterized by normal forgetfulness associated with aging. Generally, a person in this stage will self-report mild forgetfulness, particularly for names of new acquaintances and where familiar objects were left. For example, a person in this stage may think to himself or herself, "Where did I leave my glasses?" and re-trace his or her steps to find the glasses in the home. The person may still be employed, and not experience any significant changes in work performance. Furthermore, a person may only experience this forgetfulness during times of stress, fatigue, or sleeplessness. When asked, the person has appropriate concern and awareness of being forgetful at times, and quickly self-corrects during an error. Often, symptoms are not evident to family or a physician upon examination.

Activities for this Stage:

As the patient is not experiencing true therapeutic impairments at this level, structured therapy is not warranted. It is helpful to encourage persons in the very mild cognitive decline stage to engage in thirty minutes per day of cognitively stimulating new learning activities. For example, a person in this stage may find benefits in learning a new language, learning to play a new musical instrument, taking adult education courses, or learning a new needle craft.

Behavioral Problems Encountered in this Stage: No behavioral problems are typically encountered during this stage.

Mild Cognitive Communication Impairment

(Scores 5-15)

Description of this Stage:
In this stage, you may note your loved one exhibits increased forgetfulness, slight difficulty concentrating, and reduced ability to perform in the workplace. Often, this is the stage when your loved one will opt to leave the workplace due to difficulty solving complex problems due to longer processing time. A manager or colleagues may note that your loved one is less efficient in his/her typical duties. Word finding deficits begin to develop at this stage, and you may note that the person substitutes one word for another, or simply cannot think of the appropriate word quite frequently in conversation ("It is on the tip of my tongue"). When you attempt to discuss these findings, your loved one may display denial, or anxiety. He or she may use humor to attempt to conceal or deflect the deficits, or even change the subject when approached. It is wise to consult a neurologist at this stage, and consider beginning structured therapy with a speech-language pathologist or neuropsychologist if your loved one is amenable. Speech-language pathology services are covered under Medicare guidelines for cognitive communication deficits related to dementia, if your loved one is a Medicare beneficiary.

Communication Techniques for this Stage:

As word finding deficits can begin to develop during this stage, you may note changes in conversations with your loved one. Even the most articulate, educated persons may substitute words (for example, "fork" for "knife") or be unable to completely recall certain words ("It is on the tip of my tongue but I just cannot think of it"). Intervention via a speech-language pathologist can be particularly advantageous in this stage. It is critical to permit your loved one to complete his/her thought, allowing him/her adequate response time. It may be frustrating for you (the listener), but avoid interrupting or completing his/her sentences unless your loved one specifically asks for help. You may consider giving semantic "clues" to assist with specific word finding (i.e. "It is silver, sharp, serrated, and you use it to cut your steak"). By describing the item by size, color, shape, smell, noise, and/or function you evoke a multi-sensory approach to the word to stimulate recall. I find that a good sense of humor can immensely lead to communication successes at this stage. Finding fault or drawing attention to word finding deficits may lead to communication anxieties in the future, so it is best to be encouraging at this time.

Activities for this Stage:
Activities for this stage should focus on structure to compensate for errors made in activities of daily living.
- Efforts should be made to develop a graphic organizer, such as a calendar, to improve orientation to elements of date/time, and to improve recall of events. Your loved one may benefit from carrying a pocket calendar,

or utilizing an electronic calendar on a cell phone/tablet with programmed alerts for reminders. If a wall calendar is to be used in the home, it should be placed in an easily accessible, clearly visible location. Many people benefit from a calendar placed in the kitchen, as people tend to start their days in this room and can review events of the day in the morning for improved orientation.

- If your loved one is tech-savvy, alerts can be programmed for medications, birthdays, and just prior to events (i.e. leave for MD appointment alert occurring 30 minutes prior to actual appointment). Of course, in order for this to be beneficial, he/she must have his/her device with him/her, so leaving a post-it at the exit door such as "Do I have my phone?" may prove to be a sufficient reminder at this stage.
- Your loved one may benefit from making "To-Do" lists, so ensuring adequate notepads and writing instruments are available in the home is vital.
- Written instruction cards can be created to improve operation of cell phones, remote controls, smart phones, and computers. You may consider typing up instructions to check a voicemail on a cell phone, for example.
- Medication management is a concern if your loved one is living alone. If you visit weekly, consider purchasing a pill box from the pharmacy and pre-filling medications for the week. You may find you need to call and remind your loved one to take medications, or you may need to program alerts in an electronic device as previously stated.

- Furthermore, your loved one may benefit from interaction with young children or animals, such as reading them books and engaging in games, to give them a sense of purpose and control.

Behavioral Problems Encountered in this Stage:
Often behavioral problems encountered for this stage are associated with aspects of denial, or anxiety. A loved one in this stage may benefit from counseling with a mental health professional, or from medicinal interventions prescribed by a physician to reduce underlying anxiety. Your loved one may refuse to see a professional at this stage due to denial. This can be extremely frustrating for the family, and can lead to frequent quarrels about the subject. As a loved one, it is imperative at this stage to listen without blaming or criticizing the person. I find that kindness and compassion, rather than overt critiques, go much further in this stage to persuade your loved one to see a professional. You may want to present it as a trial: "if you do not like it, you do not have to return." Quality, experienced evaluating healthcare professionals have exceptional rapport building skills, and you may be pleased to find your loved one actually asking to return. Acceptance of cognitive impairment at this stage is crucial, as patients who have greater awareness of their deficits often respond better to therapy.

Moderate Cognitive Communication Impairment

(Scores 16-30)

Description of this Stage:
The Moderate Cognitive Communication Impairment Stage is vast, with a wide range of characteristics. The behaviors one may exhibit at the beginnings of this stage may differ drastically from those at the end, when your loved one is transitioning into the severe stage. Major memory deficiencies are the overall hallmark of this stage, with many loved ones unable to recall address, phone number, or elements of the date. Many persons will start to withdraw from family or friends because socialization becomes difficult. Word finding deficits will become more prevalent, sometimes creating a "language of confusion." Thus, there may be adequate grammatical structure and pitch/stress, but the content words (nouns) chosen are non-sensical, or resemble jargon. Cognitive deficits will be apparent and clear to the physician and loved ones. Traveling alone to new locations becomes nearly impossible, and the patient is now unable to manage finances independently. Your loved one may need verbal reminders to move to the next step of a task (due to difficulty sequencing events), or to simply maintain engagement in a task, such as eating.

You may find that your loved one has relatively preserved long-term memory (can remember address as a child), but poor short-term memory (cannot remember what he or she ate for breakfast that morning).

Communication Techniques for this Stage:
Meaningful communicative interactions with others may become notably impaired as this stage progresses. As a result, you may see your loved one withdraw from social situations that he/she once enjoyed. It is critical to first minimize any external environmental distractions (turn off television, silence cellular phone, speak in a quiet space) to ensure your loved one is able to focus on the communicative interaction. When speaking, present your questions or statements clearly, avoiding lengthy utterances. As this stage progresses, it can be extremely helpful to phrase questions in a yes/no format ("Would you like some eggs?" rather than "What would you like for breakfast?"). Allow your loved one ample time to respond prior to bombarding him/her with additional questions. If you are referencing a concrete, three-dimensional object and it is within reach or view, it can be beneficial to point or touch the item when discussing it to provide additional visual input. You may consider creating a very simple, written or pictorial daily schedule for your loved one to minimize behavioral problems. For example, a written or pictorial, "wake up, eat breakfast, brush teeth, get dressed, fold laundry, eat lunch, etc." may give your loved one more organization, structure, and purpose for his or her day. This structure may minimize fear or anxiety that tends to heighten during this stage. It is extremely important not to utilize "baby talk" when addressing your loved one, such as a high pitch voice or utilizing diminutives ("nana" for "banana"). This can be perceived to be disrespectful by the geriatric listener.

Activities for this Stage:

Please consider the following activities for your loved one at this stage:

- Folding clothing, towels and bed linens: *targets sequencing skills and categorization abilities*
- Sorting clothing by type of garment or color: *targets categorization by semantic qualities*
- Gross motor games such as playing catch with a ball: *targets turn-taking skills*
- Winding or unwinding yarn: *targets basic problem-solving skills*
- Promoting conversations with photo albums: *targets memory and word-finding abilities, via reminiscing through positive events that occurred in the past*
- Sorting beds by color and stringing them on yarn: *targets sequencing skills and categorization abilities*
- Setting a table for a meal: *targets sequencing skills*
- Assisting in food preparation (i.e. stirring batter with spoon, no heat or sharp objects): *targets sequencing skills*
- Dusting furniture: *targets basic problem-solving skills*
- Reminiscing with music from various decades: *targets memory, via reminiscence*
- Stuffing envelopes: *targets sequencing skills*
- Puzzles (vary in complexity as stage progresses): *targets problem-solving skills*
- Watering plants: *targets sequencing skills*
- Making the bed: *targets sequencing skills*

Behavioral Problems Encountered in this Stage:
The development of behavioral issues that may put your loved one or your family's safety at risk may occur in this stage. When you are analyzing any behavior, it can be beneficial to break it down using the "ABC" method:

A: Antecedent: an event that occurs prior to the behavior
B: Behavior: what the individual is doing
C: Consequence: an event that follows the behavior

Comprehending the antecedent events that are associated with both the occurrence and nonoccurrence of problem behavior is critical in this phase. With a grasp on the antecedents, you can modify the characteristics of a difficult situation. In other words, what is actually *causing* the behavior? What does *not cause* the behavior?

Commonly experienced behavioral problems in this phase are described in the pages to follow.

Elopement: One of the most frightening behaviors, this refers to the departure of a loved one from a home without observation or knowledge of his or her departure. Many patients who were employed for many years, or extremely task-oriented will insist they must leave for work, to pick up the children, or to run errands. This is a challenging behavior to manage, as you are attempting to balance safety while maintaining your loved one's dignity. If you are noting this behavior, it is imperative to anticipate hazards and put systems in place to keep the person safe. In the beginning of this stage, placing a "stop" or "do not enter" sign will be sufficient enough as a visual cue to deter the person from eloping. A more creative design, placing an image of a bookcase on the door will camouflage the door to disguise it as a possible exit. Also, you may consider purchasing a door alarm which triggers an extremely loud siren when a doorway is opened. Furthermore, investing in a GPS watch may increase your piece of mind as it will accurately track the locator of the wearer. Always ensure your loved one at risk of elopement is wearing some sort of identity bracelet with your contact information in case he or she does make it past an exit. If your loved one tends to wander within the home at night, ensure you have adequate night-liquids and uncluttered pathways to prevent unnecessary falls. Going for accompanied, structured walks during the daytime hours may minimize elopement and wandering around the home in the evenings. Ensuring your loved one has adequate exercise in a safe environment during daytime hours is crucial to minimize this restless behavior.

Accusatory Statements: Your loved one may begin to make false accusations against you or others. Often, these accusations involve stealing of common items, such as articles of clothing, money, or glasses. You may find your loved one perseverating on this false accusation for weeks or months at a time. It is important to validate your loved one's feelings ("I see you are feeling frustrated. I am sorry that you are feeling this way") and promptly re-direct to a new task ("How about we get these plants watered?") or an alternate, cognitively appropriate activity for this stage. Consider keeping duplicates of items the person frequently accuses others of stealing (ie glasses) to prevent further perseveration or combative behaviors.

Further, I do feel it is extremely important to not automatically assume the person with a cognitive impairment is fabricating all accusatory statements. If something sounds "fishy" to you, it is worth further investigation. There are sadly many instances of abuse towards patients with cognitive impairments.

Combative behaviors: These behaviors refer to physical aggression such as hitting, pushing, spitting, and/or kicking that may begin to occur in this stage. It is important to analyze the environment and activities that occur just prior to these behaviors, as they may help reveal the reason for said behaviors, and subsequently render an appropriate solution. For example, a person experiencing paranoia, visual or auditory hallucinations may react in a physical manner. In these cases, a physician may be able to provide medication to lessen or eliminate hallucinations/paranoia. Fear is a primary feeling associated with combative behavior. A change in schedule, caregiver, speed of care provided, and pain can contribute to feelings of fear. Removing distractions and playing light, soothing music/sounds may help to reduce fear. Further, to reduce feelings of fear, always ensure you approach your loved one from the front and move slowly towards him or her. Align your body to the person's physical level, which means you may need to sit, kneel, or squat. A positive, friendly approach goes a very long way to reduce combative behaviors.

Hallucinations: These behaviors refer to hearing, seeing, smelling, or tasting something that does not truly exist in reality. For example, your loved one may see bugs crawling up the walls that do not exist. Medication prescribed by a physician may lessen or eliminate hallucinations. It is helpful to provide the physician information about what the person saw/sensed, when the event occurred, and how long it lasted. A caregiver cannot completely prevent a hallucination, however he/she can respond in a constructive manner, so the hallucination does not lead to agitation and combative behavior. Reassurance in a calm tone of voice is an optimal way to manage hallucinations. "I can tell that you seem scared. I would be scared if I saw a lot of bugs too. I will stay here with you, and you are safe with me." Do not deny the hallucination, or scold your loved one for verbalizing the hallucination. Ensure that furniture is not casting any strange shadows that are being misinterpreted by your loved one. Also cover mirrors, as your loved one may be interpreting reflections as strangers present in the room.

Rummaging/hoarding: These behaviors refer to searching for, or carefully storing random objects. Often these behaviors are a result of fear, or loss of control. Firstly, it is important to remove poisonous or other harmful items from the physical access of someone with a penchant for rummaging. Relocate these items to a hidden, locked location if they must remain in the home. Actually restricting someone from rummaging may be impossible, so it can be quite beneficial to create an area where your loved one can safely rummage. You may want to consider placing personally meaningful objects (mementos from family vacations, awards from work, diplomas) in a "safe', easily accessible rummage area.

Many persons with cognitive impairment will hoard items to a specific area, likely a drawer or box. Once you are aware of the hiding place, check it regularly. Your loved one may be hoarding perishable items, and it will be necessary to discreetly dispose of these items for safety and hygiene purposes.

Repetitive questioning: This behavior refers to the repetition of certain utterances, such as "What time is it?" If the question is always the same, it may be beneficial to provide an easy access point to the answer. For example, providing the person with a large, digital, easy to read, wall clock or watch may minimize the need for repetitive questioning, and provides you a brief response "Look at the clock." You may consider purchasing a small dry-erase board with pertinent information and placing it near your loved one for easy reference. For example, if your loved one constantly asks "Where is my son?" you may write "SON IN BOSTON" clearly without extraneous or lengthy phrasing. For a person who is no longer reading phrases, a photo of the son in Boston may suffice. Often, repetitive questioning does arise in the topic of finances, for example "Did we pay our taxes?" You may wish to create a faux letter from the Internal Revenue Service, or the bank that states the income tax return has been received, and the refund was deposited into the bank to assuage any fears that your loved one may be experiencing.

Sundowning: This term does not refer to a particular behavior, but rather a conglomeration of behaviors that can occur in this stage. Often, you may see an exacerbation in the behaviors stated above in the late afternoon and early evening. Keeping your loved one active during day, following a structured routine, and minimizing caffeine intake in the afternoon should minimize sundowning.

Severe Cognitive Communication Impairment

(Scores 31-40)

Description of this Stage:
The Severe Cognitive Communication Impairment stage is the final phase of the cognitive decline continuum. Patients in this stage are generally minimally verbal, however some may respond with single word utterances to rote questions such as "How are you?" (your loved one may state "good" regardless of feeling), or respond to a yes/no question. It is highly unlikely that your loved one will initiate a conversation in this phase. It is possible that your loved one may not recognize you, or other familiar family members in this phase. While the person is generally unaware of his or her surroundings, he or she may be able to distinguish familiar from unfamiliar persons. Cognitive deficits will be clear to physician, loved ones, and unfamiliar persons. Lethargy is common in this phase (your loved one may be bed-bound), as well as incontinence of both bladder and bowels.

A more complex complication during this phase is dysphagia, difficulty swallowing. Details regarding dysphagia management for a person with severe cognitive communication impairments are provided in the next chapter.

Communication Techniques for this Stage:
Many people assume that because their loved one is non-verbal, that he or she is non-communicative. This is completely erroneous. Facial expressions, gestures, and body language are types of communication that provide us insight to a person's inner wants and needs. It is imperative for a caregiver to have the ability to correctly interpret these non-verbal behaviors to appropriately care for a loved one. For example, consistent grimacing just prior to urination may indicate pain during the passage of urine. This may be indicative of a urinary tract infection which requires prompt treatment by a physician.

An alternative communicative technique is Intensive Interaction. This is a highly researched method in which a caregiver mirrors or copies behaviors of a loved one to initiate an interaction. For example, your loved one constantly taps his index finger on an arm of a chair, never making eye contact with you. If you mirror the behavior (you tap your index finger on the arm of a chair), your loved one may be more likely to make eye contact with you, and feel comforted by an interaction. This may lessen behavioral problems encountered during this stage as delineated below.

Activities for this Stage:
Please consider the following activities for your loved one at this stage:
- Sanding wood: *repetitive motion that provides calming input*
- Pushing a mop or broom: *repetitive motion that provides calming input*

- Hand-clapping to music: *repetitive motion integrated with auditory input*
- Rubbing lotion or scented oils on extremities: *provides tactile and sensory input*
- Providing a doll or stuffed animal: *a safe object for tactile input and comfort*
- Touching fabrics of different textures (silk, velvet, cotton): *tactile input of varying textures*
- Holding a cat or dog: *tactile input, comfort*
- Watching a fish tank or a bird feeder: *provides visual, calming input*
- Hugging: *provides deep pressure stimulation for calming input*
- Playing gentle music or a sound machine: *provides calming, auditory input*

Behavioral Problems Encountered in this Stage:

Crying/Moaning/Yelling: With the absence of verbalization, verbal output in this phase may be primarily vocalizations such as cries, moans, or shouts. These vocalizations are typically communicative attempts to indicate an unmet need. The most common unmet needs are hunger, thirst, pain relief, or environmental concerns (too hot, cold, dark, light, loud). Ensuring your loved one is receiving adequate nutrition and hydration, as well as pristine oral care may minimize these behaviors. Attempt to keep the temperature of the room suitable to the person's preferences prior to the cognitive decline. Playing soothing music or utilizing a sound machine may reduce these behaviors.

Hitting/Resistance to Care: This can be a particularly difficult behavior to manage for caregivers. After ensuring the hierarchy of needs is met, ensure you or the designated caregiver approaches your loved one in a positive manner, from the front, speaking slowly and calmly. Consider providing safe objects for your loved one to hold during care (such as a stuffed animal). During transfers (i.e. moving from supine to sit, transitioning from bed to chair), ensure a caregiver is moving slowly, allowing your loved one ample time to respond to postural changes during these transfers.

Speaking to Children about Dementia

Coping with your loved one's diagnosis is certainly difficult for the adults in the family, but it poses unique challenges for our younger family members. Often, many adults initially attempt to shield or protect their children from interacting with the person with dementia, but this is typically not the best approach.

Many children do worry that dementia is a disease that is "contagious" as they have been inclined to associate the term 'sick' with 'contagious.' Thus, it is imperative to have an honest conversation, tailored to the children's age level, about changes seen in their loved one (often a grandparent or great-grandparent). For example, you may say, "When you are sick, you get a cold or a cough, but sometimes when grandparents are sick, it changes how their brains work. Grandma's brain is changing. She can remember how much she loves us, but she has trouble remembering names for things now." Also, many children are inclined to think that if one is sick, then one will "get better" or link medication to improvement in health status. While upsetting, it is important to address that there is no medicine or cure for dementia.

If your loved one is residing in a facility, and the facility permits children during visiting hours, please bring them. You may not only provide joy to your loved one, but to other residents as well. Please just ensure that you do not leave your child unsupervised with your loved one or another resident, as behavior patterns in dementia can rapidly fluctuate. While another resident may appear to be calm and friendly, these traits may be superficial and transient.

It is also advised to openly state how *you* feel about this diagnosis. Please be open and tell your child that you are frustrated, confused, saddened, for example, as it will encourage in the open sharing of feelings.

It may be helpful to work on a family tree activity, or a family scrapbooking activity to promote awareness of the family as a whole. If your child enjoys arts and crafts, he or she may find pleasure in drawing pictures or cards for your loved one. Furthermore, there are some commercially available picture books written on the topic that you may find beneficial in sharing with your child:

Grandma's Box of Memories Helping Grandma to Remember by Jean Demetris
When My Grammy Forgets, I Remember by Toby Harberkorn
Grandpa Sea Shells by Jo Johnson
Always My Grandpa by Linda Scacco

If your child is exhibiting severe difficulties in coping with the dementia diagnosis, please consider speaking with your child's pediatrician. He or she may refer you to a child psychologist or social worker for an evaluation to determine if therapy is warranted.

Managing Your Loved One's Medical Care

There will likely come a point when your loved one will no longer be capable of managing his or her medical care. He or she may rely on you to communicate with physicians and other members of the medical team. Please consider the following points when coordinating care:

- Choose *one* primary care provider.

    Often, in this current state of medicine, when one reaches an advanced age he/she sees multiple physicians of varying specialties at a number of different facilities. While it is imperative to see specialists for consultations, it is extremely important to have a primary care provider to which all specialists report. He or she must be willing to coordinate your overall care, ensuring he or she is aware of what other medications alternate physicians may be prescribing. Ideally, a primary care provider is board certified in internal medicine, family medicine and/or geriatrics. What is the difference?

Internal Medicine: This physician has completed four years of medical school, plus a three-year residency in internal medicine. This provider is concerned with the prevention, diagnosis, and treatment of disease in those over eighteen years old.

Family Medicine: This physician has completed four years of medical school, plus a three-year residency in family medicine. This provider is concerned with prevention, diagnosis, and treatment of disease for the whole family, including pediatrics and OB/GYN care.

Geriatrics: This physician has completed four years of medical school, a three- year residency typically in internal medicine or family medicine, and an additional one-year fellowship in geriatrics. This provider is concerned with prevention, diagnosis, and treatment of disease in older adults, with further training in the aging process. This professional has immense insight regarding cognitive impairments in the aging population.

- Medication Review

Once you have chosen a primary care physician, he or she should conduct a thorough review of all medications (both prescription and over-the-counter) that your loved one is taking. It is best to bring the actual medication bottles/boxes along to the visit so the physician can easily read the dosage and instructions proposed by the specialists. The physician will review all of the medications for suitability, contraindications, and side effects. Ensure that you have a clear understanding of the medication's purpose, how it is to be taken, and the proper dosage.

- Preparation for Appointments

In addition to bringing along medications, it is also wise to write down any questions you may have in advance, leaving adequate room in between the questions to jot down pertinent answers. While the internet is an information-rich resource for research, a Google search does not replace medical school, residency, and years of experience. Also, ensure you have a list of specialists your loved one has seen recently. Most physicians will greatly appreciate the concern you show for your loved one.

Special Consideration: Dysphagia in Cognitive Impairment

Thus far we have addressed the cognitive communication concerns associated with dementia, however, it is critical to discuss the presence of swallowing disorders that can occur in this population, known as dysphagia.

Professionals assess three different phases of the swallow: oral, pharyngeal, and esophageal.

Oral Phase: The oral phase of the swallow involves sensory recognition of the food first entering the mouth, stripping food from a spoon or liquids from cup/spout/spoon, salivation, containing the food and/or liquid within the mouth, moving the food from the front to the back of the mouth (anterior-posterior transit), mastication, and ensuring there is no significant residue along the walls of the cheeks or tongue after the food or liquid is swallowed.

Pharyngeal Phase: The pharyngeal phase of the swallow is the actual "swallow" as you are thinking: the larynx elevates, the vocal folds come together, and the epiglottis retroflexes to protect food/liquid from entering the trachea into the lungs.

Esophageal Phase: The esophageal phase of the swallow refers to the food passing into the esophagus to the stomach via peristalsis, muscle contractions that are wave-like which help to propel the food or liquid.

Dysphagia can occur in one phase, two phases, or all three phases with differing severities. For example, your loved one may have significant difficulty moving food from the front of the mouth to the back of the mouth in a timely fashion ("holding" food in his or her mouth), but once a swallow is triggered, it moves smoothly to the stomach without difficulty. Due to the nuances and complexity, it is critical that a professional is consulted when one with dementia is having difficulty with any stage of swallow. Typically, dysphagia is more associated with advanced cognitive impairments, but it can occur at any phase in the continuum.

As a caregiver, you play an instrumental role in managing your loved one's dysphagia, from recognizing concerning symptoms to management via diet modifications, and other strategies discussed below. As pneumonia due to dysphagia accounts for nearly 70% of causes of death for patients with Alzheimer's, it is imperative to be aware of assessment and management options for your loved one.

Signs and symptoms of dysphagia
One does not have to demonstrate all of the symptoms below, however these signs are typically associated with dysphagia:
- Coughing during or immediately after a meal
- A "wet" voice during or immediately after a meal (sounds gurgly), which may be more pronounced when your loved one consumes liquids
- Holding foods in the mouth for a prolonged period of time
- Facial color changes
- Frequent, recurrent pneumonias
- Becoming fatigued as a meal progresses

- Weight loss
- Drooling

If you note any of the symptoms above, please notify your primary care physician or neurologist immediately. He or she will refer you to a speech-language pathologist, who is the most qualified professional to assess and treat swallowing disorders occurring due to dementia.

Assessment of Swallowing Disorders

The assessment of swallowing disorders is truly a book of its own! Below, please find commonly ordered assessments of swallowing, and a brief description of each.

Bedside swallow assessment: If your loved one resides in a facility, and the staff become concerned regarding his or her ability to swallow, typically a speech-language pathologist is consulted for a Bedside Swallow Assessment. A speech-language pathologist will evaluate your loved one's teeth, lips, jaw, tongue, cheeks, and palate, as well as ask specific questions to your family regarding the nature of the swallowing problem. The SLP will observe your loved one swallow a variety of substances (typically liquids and solids of varying texture), checking for signs of dysphagia and aspiration.

Modified Barium Swallow/Videofluoroscopy: During this x-ray, your loved one will be asked to ingest a barium solution, and consume food products that are coated in barium. It is performed by a speech-language pathologist, in conjunction with a radiologist to examine the oral, pharyngeal, and esophageal phase of swallow. This test allows the professional to determine the specific cause and location of swallowing difficulty.

Fiber-optic Endoscopic Swallow Evaluation: A speech-language pathologist, often in conjunction with an otolaryngologist, will examine the pharynx with a special camera as you consume food and beverages coated with food coloring.

Esophagram/Barium Swallow: Similar to a Modified Barium Swallow (it is an x-ray during which one ingests liquid barium), this test is not performed by a speech-language pathologist, and it examines the esophagus, stomach and the duodenum.

Esophageal manometry: A small tube is inserted into the esophagus typically by a gastroenterologist, which is connected to a pressure recorder to measure the muscular contractions of the esophagus as your loved one swallows.

Managing Swallowing Disorders

Subsequent to a comprehensive swallow evaluation, a speech-language pathologist will design a personalized treatment plan to improve your loved one's swallow function. The following management techniques are meant to be a general guide. Please heed the specific recommendations provided to you by a medical professional.

Environmental Modifications
- Reduce distractions during mealtime. Serve food in a quiet environment, away from the television or constantly ringing phones.
- Focus on color contrast between the plate to the placement, and the food to the plate. Mashed potatoes on a white plate, served on a white placement with a white tablecloth will not help your loved one visually discriminate! Research has indicated that food served

on red plates to patients with Alzheimer's improved intake by twenty-five percent.
- Consider serving hot cereal or soup in a mug (with an adequate handle) to improve intake.
- Avoid introducing unfamiliar routines. A loved one who never ate breakfast for the first eighty years of his or her life, probably will not want to start eating breakfast at eighty-one!
- Encourage a calm, comfortable environment that is not rushed.

Body Positioning
- Ensure your loved one is sitting upright, as close to ninety degrees as possible. It is preferable that your loved one is out of bed, sitting in a chair for meals.
- Place fork/spoon in the dominant hand at the beginning of the meal.
- Encourage upright positioning for at least forty-five minutes after meal time to ensure all food is passed into the stomach. This is particularly important for those with acid reflux.

Safe Swallow Strategies
- Only serve meals to your loved one when he or she is awake and alert. Serving food to someone who is drowsy or lethargic is extremely dangerous.
- Alternate between solids and liquids. If you are feeding your loved one, feed two-three fork/spoonfuls, followed by a sip of liquid. Ensure your rate is slow.
- Do not continue to feed your loved one if you note food/liquid still in the mouth from the previous

forkful/sip. Encourage your loved one to first swallow before administering any additional food or drink.
- Ensure your loved one has adequate dental care. Make sure that dentures fit appropriately (if applicable). A non-verbal patient with dementia may not be able to express tooth/gum pain, but lack of appetite may be due to dental issues.

Diet Modification
If the above conditions are satisfied, and your loved one still exhibits continued difficulty consuming food or liquid, a speech-language pathologist may consider changing the texture of the food or liquid to reduce aspiration risk or improve overall intake. If intake amount is concerning, a registered dietitian may be able to recommend a specific diet plan to improve overall intake, or specific nutritional supplements. A physician may prescribe an appetite stimulant to further increase intake.

How can a diet be modified?
Both solids and liquids can be changed to reduce dysphagia-associated risks. Below please find common texture modifications that may be recommended to you by a speech-language pathologist.

Solid Modifications

<u>Soft solids</u>: A nearly regular diet, this diet excludes very hard, sticky or exceptionally crunchy solids. For example, foods such as nuts, dried fruit, chewy candies, and chunky peanut butter would be excluded in this texture.

Mechanical Soft solids: Most foods can be included in this diet, as long as they are cooked and chopped. Soft bread is sometimes included in this diet category (will be evaluated by the speech-language pathologist). The key specifications are that meats and vegetables must be chopped into ¼ inch pieces.

Ground solids: This diet is similar to the mechanical soft diet, however all meats in this category must be ground and typically bread is not permitted.

Puree solids: This diet contains foods that do not require any mastication, such as mashed potatoes or pudding. Solid foods may be blended with water or broth to create nutritionally dense puree solids. Molds are available to form puree foods into shapes resembling solid foods.

Blenderized solids: Very similar to the puree diet, this diet has more a more watery or brothy content. For example, watery applesauce would fit in this category.

Liquid Modifications

Liquids can be modified via special thickening agents that are readily available at local pharmacies, or these liquids can be purchased from specialty stores pre-thickened. The agents' thickening ability do differ, and each container will indicate specific directions for mixing. Your speech-language pathologist should train you and your family in thickening liquids to the appropriate indicated level. It will take some practice initially- you might end up with cement-like water the first time around!

Nectar-thick liquids: These liquids are slightly thicker than water. They do not taste like nectar, refer to fruit nectar, or contain nectar. The name is referring to the thickness level.

<u>Honey-thick liquids</u>: These liquids are as thick as honey. They do not taste like honey, and they do not contain any honey, the name is referring to the thickness level.

<u>Pudding-thick liquids</u>: These liquids are as thick as pudding. They do not taste like pudding and they do not contain any pudding, the name is referring to the thickness level. These liquids provide minimal hydration, and it is quite easy to become dehydrated on this diet. Please discuss hydration concerns with a medical professional if this diet is recommended.

Improving Intake

Taste/Temperature Modifications
Altering the taste or temperature of both solids and liquids may improve overall intake. Taste sensation does diminish as we age, so elderly loved ones may crave intensely flavored foods, such as sweets. Appetite preferences may change over time due to evolving taste sensation. A dietician can assist you to choose sweet foods that do have some nutritional value, such as a vitamin-fortified milkshake. And of course, always check the temperature of food and drinks prior to offering it to your loved one.

Verbal Encouragement
A little verbal encouragement can go a long way! You may need to be creative in your suggestions. A non-obtrusive way to coax a person to improve intake is to say something like, "I have a new recipe I want to cook for my husband. Would you please try it and tell me what you think?"

Appetite Stimulants
If the above suggestions have been implemented, and found ineffective, you may want to speak to your loved one's primary care physician about appetite stimulants. There are a variety of available prescription medications that do stimulate one's appetite, however their benefit-to-risk ratio must be carefully considered by the physician. These medications do have side effects that must be examined and evaluated.

Oral Hygiene
We often underestimate the importance of oral hygiene; however, it is critical in the geriatric population. Please ensure your loved one's mouth is clean after a meal. There should be no residual food or liquid on the tongue, in the cheeks, or on the surface of the teeth. The best practice is to brush one's teeth after each meal, paying particular attention to the oral care after the evening meal. You may consider purchasing a water-flosser to provide a strong stream of water to clean the mouth. As one typically lays supine (on one's back) while sleeping, this position can allow for any particles still in the mouth to be aspirated. It is extremely important to assist your loved one in thorough oral care.

End of Life Discussions Regarding Non-Oral Feeding

As the dementia progresses, your loved one may have very minimal intake of food and liquid. He or she may be very lethargic or may be sleeping most of the day and night. When a person reaches these advanced stages, you may be confronted with a decision to insert a feeding tube for artificial nutrition or hydration. This is a controversial issue in medicine, and it does have ethical conundrums as well.

First, it is wise to have these discussions when your loved one is in the early stages of the disease process, when he or she is still competent to complete advanced directives or a living will, a legal document that delineates one's specific, future medical care decisions. In this document, your loved one may specifically address concerns regarding tube feeding, mechanical ventilation, dialysis, and organ donation. He or she may also name a "health care proxy" or "power of attorney", a person who is appointed to make medical decisions in the event that he or she is not competent or unable to do so. While this continues to be a very challenging topic, having the foresight to have these conversations early in the disease process is key.

Without appropriate nutrition or hydration, the human body stimulates endorphins, natural substances that are produced to naturally reduce pain. In coordination with drugs such as morphine, a physician (specifically one who specializes in palliative care), may be able to eliminate any pain with these end stages of life.

Research shows that tube-feeding in the dementia population shows no significant benefit. Artificial tube feeding does not serve to lower the incidence of aspiration pneumonia, and there is no evidence that it will prolong one's life in this population (Friedrich, 2013). Artificial feeding in isolation also denies a person the joy of tasting food/beverages, and limits the social interaction that mealtime often brings. Furthermore, tubes/insertion sites can become infected, leading to additional problems and complications requiring antibiotic treatment. Often if residing in a facility, your loved one's upper extremities will be restrained to deter him or her from pulling out the tube. It is critical that you speak to the medical team regarding benefits and risks of tube feeding for your loved one's specific situation. I believe firmly in hand-feeding (oral feeding) to preserve the patient's quality of life, comfort, and social interaction, even if the amount of food accepted is minimal.

References

Darnell, O. (n.d.). *A Room Without Doors* [pamphlet]. N.P.: n.p.

Friedrich, L. (2013). End-of-life nutrition: is tube feeding the solution? *Annals of Long-Term Care: Clinical Care and Aging.* 21, 30-33.

Made in United States
North Haven, CT
04 January 2023

30586993R00030